All You Wanted To Know About
Hatha Yoga

Ravindra Kumar, Ph.D.
(Swami Atmananda)

New Dawn

NEW DAWN
a division of Sterling Publishers (P) Ltd.
A-59, Okhla Industrial Area, Phase-II, New Delhi-110020
Tel : 6916209, 6916165, 6912677, 6910050
E-mail : ghai@nde.vsnl.net.in
www.sterlingpublishers.com

All You Wanted to Know About - Hatha Yoga
© 2000, Sterling Publishers Private Limited
ISBN 81 207 2325 2
Reprint 2002

All rights are reserved. No part of this publication may be reproduced, stored in a retrieval system or transmitted, in any form or by any means, mechanical, photocopying, recording or otherwise, without prior written permission of the publisher.

Published by Sterling Publishers Pvt. Ltd., New Delhi-110020.
Lasertypeset by Vikas Compographics, New Delhi-110020.
Printed at Shagun Offset, New Delhi-110029.

Contents

Preface	5
Introduction	7
1. Preliminaries	10
2. Padmasana	14
3. Siddhasana	19
4. Bhujangasana	24
5. Dhanurasana	28
6. Vajrasana	32
7. Ardhamatsyendrasana	38
8. Padapashchimottasana	42
9. Gorakshasana	47
10. Yogamudrasana	50
11. Sarvangasana	53

12. Katipindmardanasana 57
13. Mayurasana 60
14. Halasana 63
15. Chakrasana 67
16. Shavasana 70
17. Three locks (tribandh) 75
18. Three Purifications 82
19. Integral Path in Modern Age 88
20. Special Postures 134
21. Postures for Menstruation 149
22. General Advice 159

Preface

Hatha Yoga is a marvellous means of exercising, stretching, and purifying the body so as to make it healthy, and a vital instrument of the mind and soul. In Sanskrit, *ha* means the sun, *tha* means the moon. It is, therefore, a practice of harmonising the body's currents (feeling, thinking, willing, and acting) until they are in perfect balance. The awareness is raised to the level of the superconscious state.

The book presents the elements of Hatha Yoga in a simple and short way for those who have no time to go into rigorous studies. It is based on my own practice and personal experiences with *Kundalini*, while laying the foundations of the Academy of Kundalini Yoga and Quantum Soul at New Delhi, Copenhagen, Florida and London.

Thanks are also due to Jytte Kumar Larsen for providing computing facilities and related help.

Swami Atmananda (Ravindra Kumar, PhD)
Founder President
Academy of Kundalini Yoga and Quantum Soul
58-61 Vashisht Park, Pankha Road,
New Delhi-110046
Tel: 5047091, 5041368, 5034143, 5137567

Introduction

The *Vedas* advocated three different paths for the search of Truth — knowing the Self or *Atma: Bhakti Yoga*, the path of devotion for those whose heart is more developed than the mind; *Jnana Yoga*, the path of knowledge for those whose mind is more developed than the heart; *Karma Yoga*, the path of selfless action for those who have their heart and mind more or less equally developed. In the medieval ages, the yogis of the Nath sect thought that there would be people who would have neither the heart nor the mind reasonably developed. So how should such people know the Self? Guru Gorakh Nath and others thus created Hatha Yoga, the path of austerity for people to begin searching for Truth from scratch.

The word "yoga" is derived from the Sanskrit root *yuj* which means "harnessing horses to the chariot." This, therefore, is the preparation for liberating oneself from the clutches of the five physical senses and putting oneself on the path of divine reality. It began with experiential and non-intellectual practices in the past; but today, however, it has developed into a deep philosophy.

Hatha Yoga is the most popular form of yoga today, especially in the West, but more often than not, it is mainly practised for health and vitality only. However, few dedicated men and women unite finite life with infinite life and live in abundant well-being and universal harmony. This book deals with the subject of physical well-being and freedom at large, and yet paves the way towards the higher goal of self-realisation.

Preliminaries

Ordinary people do not make attempts at reviving their dormant energies and continue living an insignificant life. Yogic postures called *asanas* help you revive these dormant energies. With regular practice you attain a healthy body, happy state of mind and sharp intellect. The *rishis* observed the *asanas*, in which a yogi automatically awakens the dormant powers, for several millennia. Then they prescribed the converse; that is, if a person regularly practises these asanas, his/her dormant energies can be awakened. And in course of time these asanas were duly respected by people round the world. The book contains the keys to make you a better person and also to make your life an extraordinary one.

Rules to be observed

- The asanas should be practised on an empty stomach or after 3½ hours of a heavy meal or after 1½ hours of a light meal.
- One should inhale through the nose and never through the mouth.
- To retain the electric currents generated by the asanas one

should practise on a cushion made of wool or any other material which is a bad conductor.
- The practice has to be rhythmic and not by force as the asanas are not athletic exercises.
- One should inhale before the start of an asana, retain the breath during the asana, and exhale after the asana is over.
- One should wear loose garments during the practice.
- A bath or shower should be taken after some time of the asanas and one should avoid going to cold or windy places soon afterwards.

- Keep inhaling and exhaling in-between the asanas to relieve the tension in various parts of the body.
- Urination soon after the asanas flushes out the harmful elements collected during the practice.
- Drinking some water afterwards helps in the removal of dirt collected in the joints.
- Female practitioners should avoid the practice of asanas during pregnancy and menstruation.

Padmasana

Method
- Sit down on a cushion.
- While exhaling, turn the right foot and place it on the left thigh. Turn the left foot and place it on the right thigh. The roles of left and right feet can be reversed, according to one's convenience.
- The soles should be facing upwards, the heels downwards and the knees should be touching the ground. Head, neck, breast and the spinal cord should be straight and averagely tight.

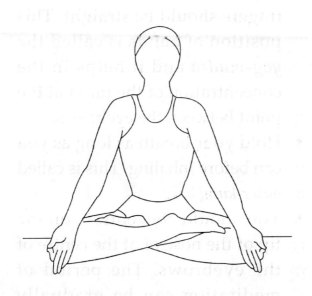

Padmasana

- Both hands should be placed on the knees with the thumb making a circular posture with the first finger while the remaining three fingers should be straight. This position of hands is called the *yog-mudra* and it helps in the concentration of the mind at the point between the eyebrows.
- Hold your breath as long as you can before inhaling. This is called *outer-kumbhak*.
- You should concentrate on the tip of the nose or at the centre of the eyebrows. The period of meditation can be gradually increased from one minute to one

hour, increasing by one minute every third day.

During this posture, one is conscious of the fact that the energy which is lying dormant at the base of the spine is gradually waking up. You should keep inhaling deeply, retaining your breath as long as you can (called *inner-kumbhak*), and then exhale slowly.

Benefits

Several diseases gradually disappear and you become more cheerful and zealous, there is lustre on the face, intellect becomes sharp, negative thoughts are suppressed while positive and good thoughts take over, the mind becomes calm and retention of semen is achieved. It becomes easier to give up the use of intoxicants.

Blood related diseases, indigestion, insomnia, arthritis, impotence and extra fat begin to disappear. Capacity to work increases tremendously and you do not tire easily.

Regular practise of the asana helps in the awakening of the *Kundalini* (dormant serpent power) which breaks the chain of death and rebirth once and for all.

Siddhasana

Next to padmasana, but no lesser in benefit, rather an alternative to Padmasana, is *siddhasana*. The literal meaning of siddhasana is "the posture of accomplishment". It is the best among asanas and is very dear to yogis. One should dedicate oneself for the perfection of siddhasana.

Method
- Sit comfortably on the cushion. Press the heel of the left foot against the mid-point between the anus and the genitals, called

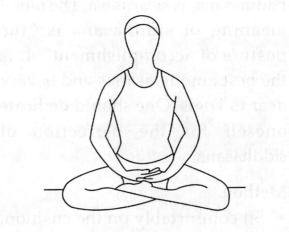

Siddhasana

the *root-centre* or *mooladhara-chakra.*

- Press the heel of the right foot against the pelvic bone just above the genitals, taking care that the genitals are not crushed. The heels of both the feet should be at the centre of the thighs.
- Keep both the palms one above the other at the centre, or keep the hands in yogamudra as in padmasana.
- Eyes can be kept open or closed and respiration should be deep and natural. Concentrate on the point between the eyebrows (*ajna-chakra*). However, there should be a continuous

awareness of the pressure on the perennial trigger point.
- It is good to point out here that the root centre and eyebrow centre are internally connected to each other through nerves, and the awakening of one affects the other automatically.
- The time can be gradually increased from five minutes to several hours.
- In the case of women, the lower heel is placed just inside the entrance to the vagina while the upper heel presses against the clitoris. Some people call it *siddha-yoni-asana*. Other details

are the same as in siddhasana for men.

Benefits

Nearly the same as in padmasana. Besides, it is especially good to achieve celibacy since the flow of seminal fluid is ultimately reversed, *kundalini* is awakened and, one is liberated from the clutches of body and mind.

The process can be expedited with the use of *tribandh* (discussed later). Success of this single asana can break the chain of incarnations on the earth. Perfect health and freedom from diseases are automatic by-products.

Bhujangasana

The literal meaning of *bhujangasana* is "the posture in the form of the hood of a cobra".

Method
- Lie down on the cushion with your face down. Join the feet together.
- Keep the palms parallel to the shoulders.
- Raise your torso and head up such that you look at the sky, focussing your attention on the centre of the throat.

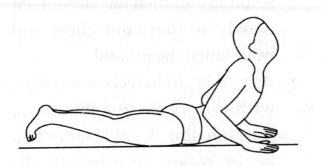

Bhujangasana

- Take care that your navel touches the ground. Feel the pressure at the lower end of the spine. Remain in the posture for 20 seconds and then lower yourself slowly so that your chest and head touch the ground.
- As you begin to feel comfortable with this asana in a few days, start inhaling deeply before you begin, retain your breath all-through for 20 seconds, and then exhale slowly as you lower your body. One can practise this posture 8 to 10 times every day.

Benefits

It cures indigestion and most diseases, and awakens the *kundalini*. It is good for strengthening the spinal column and in removing all kinds of related problems. The nervous system is cleansed and strengthened. Menstruation is regularised in ladies. Cough-related diseases are cured.

Dhanurasana

Dhanurasana is "the posture in the form of a bow".

Method
- Lie down on the cushion with your face down.
- Join your legs and bend them at the knees.
- Take your hands backwards and hold your leg by the ankles.
- Exhale and pull the feet so that a bow is formed. Bend your head backwards and look towards the sky.

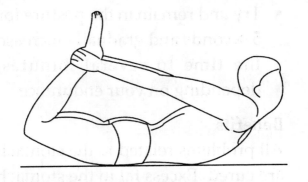

Dhanurasana

- Let your body rest on the stomach, specially on the navel.
- Inhale before beginning the asana, hold your breath during the posture, and exhale slowly at the end.
- Try and remain in the posture for 5 seconds and gradually increase the time to several minutes, depending on your endurance.

Benefits

All problems related to the stomach are cured. Excess fat in the stomach is reduced, the heart and neck become strong, eye-sight improves, and the face and body becomes graceful.

Digestion and appetite are improved and diseases related to the womb and menstruation irregularities in women are cured.

Vajrasana

The literal meaning of this word is "the posture strong like steel".

Method
- Bend the legs at the knees and sit on the heels making a comfortable seat of the heels.
- The toes should touch each other and the heels should support the hips.
- Keep your waist and back straight and let your hands rest on the two knees.

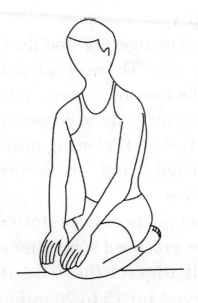

Vajrasana

- Concentrate on the point between the eye-brows. The posture should be held for 10 to 30 minutes.

Benefits

It helps in digestion and the nerves gain power. The main advantage is that the flow of semen is reversed, causing the body to become strong like steel. A flickering mind gets stabilised and concentration improves.

This is the only posture which can be practised soon after meals, and it digests the food if it is observed for 15 to 20 minutes. It makes one smart and cheerful.

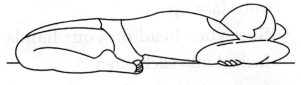

Suptavajrasana

It provides protection from most diseases. In women, irregularities in menstruation is cured.
- An extension of vajrasana is the suptavajrasana in which you sit in vajrasana and then you fall on your back on the ground with your face up.
- Rest your head on your hands locked into each other.
- Concentrate on the root centre, below the spinal column.

Benefits

The main advantage of this asana is that the central nerve or *sushumna* opens up with regular practice, and the path of the *kundalini* is thus cleared.

In general, advantages of the basic asana which is the vajrasana, are multiplied. All the knots connected with the various *chakras* get strengthened.

Ardhamatsyendrasana

The creator of this posture is Guru Matsyendranath of the medieval age.

Method
- Sit on a cushion and stretch your legs.
- Bend the left leg at the knee and place the heel under the anus region. The left heel should touch the right thigh.
- Now bend the right leg at the knee. Take it to the other side of the left leg and place it on the ground.

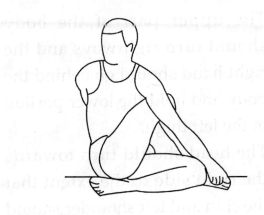

Ardhamatsyendrasana

- Now the left hand should cross the right leg on its opposite side and hold the toe of the right leg with the left hand.
- The upper part of the body should turn rightways and the right hand should go behind the body and hold the lower portion of the left thigh.
- The head should turn towards the right side to the extent that the chin and left shoulder should be in one straight line.
- The chest should be stretched straight. The attention should be concentrated at the navel.

- In the beginning, remain in this posture for 5 seconds and then gradually increase it to 1 minute.

Benefits

It gives a twist to the spinal column which is the best exercise for strengthening the spine and invigorating the body.

Nerves related to the spine, back, neck and the area below the navel region are also exercised. Appetite increases too.

Padapashchimottasana

It is supposed to be a complete asana according to Lord Shiva in *Shivasanhita*. Not everyone can master this posture; those who can, attain perfect health and can awaken the *kundalini* through the practise of this single posture. The same is true about padmasana and siddhasana. Each one of these asanas is complete in itself.

Method
- Stretch your legs on the cushion. The thighs, knees and toes

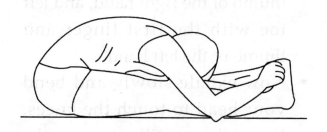

Padapashchimottasana

should be joined together and should be placed firmly on the ground.
- Stretch the hands and hold the right toe with the first finger and thumb of the right hand, and left toe with the first finger and thumb of the left hand.
- Now exhale slowly and bend your head to touch the knees. Your elbows will go across the knees and touch the ground.
- Having exhaled completely, hold your breath and concentrate on the navel centre.

- One can begin by remaining in the pose for 30 seconds and then increase the time to 15 to 20 minutes gradually.

Benefits

The door of the central nerve *sushumna* opens up and *prana* (life force) travelling through the spinal column awakens the *bindu centre* (point between the eyebrow centre and the crown centre). This leads to the flow of nectar which rejuvenates the whole body and leads one into *samadhi*.

Victory over sex is one essential step before liberation and it is this single posture which provides for this requirement.

The whole body being rejuvenated, most of the common diseases are eliminated, flow of semen is reversed, indigestion and insomnia are cured, and tranquillity of mind is achieved. Guru Gorakh Nath of the medieval age was responsible for highlighting this posture for the upliftment of humanity in general.

Gorakshasana

Method
- Sit cross legged on a cushion and bring your heels together.
- Hold them in the cup of your palms, and pull the heels towards the body to touch and press against it, if possible.
- Inhale deeply while beginning the asana and hold the breath as long as you can, and press your chin against the body. Concentrate on the root centre below the base of the spine.

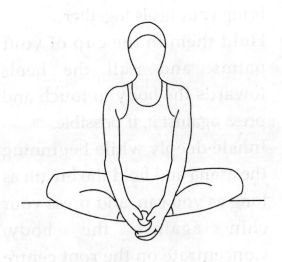

Gorakshasana

- The time can be gradually increased upto 10 minutes or more.

Benefits

Your legs become stronger. The body becomes thin and strong, and intellect sharpens.

It brings a sense of tranquillity to mind, develops intuition, improves digestion, rids one of diseases. You begin to remain cheerful. It also helps in the awakening of the *kundalini*.

Yogamudrasana

Method
- Sit in padmasana. Put your hands behind your back and hold one hand with the other.
- Pull your hands towards the waist and spine.
- Exhale and bend the body towards the ground until your head touches the ground.
- Now slowly straighten the body and inhale.
- One can also practise this posture in sukhasana or siddhasana but

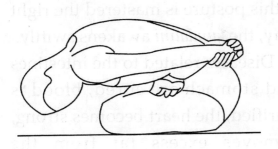

Yogamudrasana

maximum benefits are achieved in padmasana. The period of the asana should normally be 3 minutes.

Benefits

If this posture is mastered the right way, the *kundalini* awakens swiftly.

Diseases related to the intestines and stomach are cured, blood is purified, the heart becomes strong, removes excess fat from the abdomen, the body becomes strong and the capacity to work increases.

Sarvangasana

Method
- Lie down on the cushion. Exhale and raise the whole body upwards while keeping the legs together and straight.
- Hold the body erect keeping the palms of both the hands at the waist.
- The elbows should be kept on the ground and the whole body should rest on the shoulders and neck.
- The chin should touch and press against the chest. Concentrate on

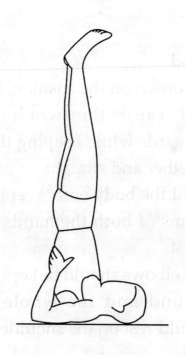

Sarvangasana

the toes or at the throat centre, keeping your eyes closed.
- Now inhale and keep the respiration normal. The time should normally be three to five minutes, although a veteran can take it to several hours.

Benefits

Reversal of the seminal fluid, improvement in appetite, tightness of the skin, rejuvenation, and strengthening of the thyroid gland in particular are some of the advantages.

Although head-stand is the proper posture but it has several side effects and ill-effects due to improper practice which this posture does not have. And, all benefits of head-stand are available through sarvangasana and padapaschimottasana. There are several other benefits such as regulation of menstruation in women, improved eye sight and sharpening of the intellect.

Katipindmardanasana

The literal meaning of this word is "the posture that presses the urinary region".

Method
- Lie on the cushion with your face up.
- Spread your hands to the sides and close the fists.
- Bend your legs in such a way that the knee of the left leg touches the heel of the right leg, while the head is turned rightwards.
- Inhale before beginning this asana, hold the breath during this

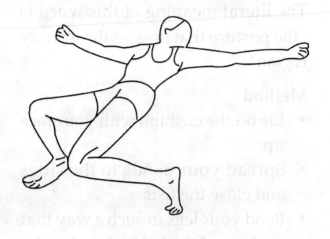

Katipindmardanasana

posture as long as you can, and concentrate on the root centre, which is a point below the spine.
- Now reverse the role of left and right parts of the body. The whole process can be carried out 15 to 20 times.

Benefits

It is the best posture to remove stones from the gall bladder. The stone breaks into pieces and is flushed out with the urine.

All diseases related to the urinary system, such as pain in the waist, stiffness of the back-bone, diabetes, impotence, cystitis, formation of gas, indigestion, etc., are cured with regular practise of this asana.

Mayurasana

The literal meaning of this word is "the posture in the form of a peacock".

Method
- Bend your knees and sit on the cushion.
- Place your palms on the ground with the fingers facing the direction of the feet and joined together.
- Bend the hand at the elbows and place them around the navel.

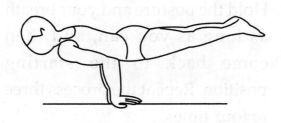

Mayurasana

- Now exhale and raise your feet above the ground, keeping them straight.
- Let your head down so that the whole body is parallel to the ground.
- Concentrate on the navel centre. Hold the posture and your breath as long as you can, and then come back to the starting position. Repeat the process three to four times.

Benefits

The digestive system is worked up making it strong, and it helps in the observance of celibacy.

Halasana

Method
- Lie down on a cushion with your hands at the sides.
- Now exhale and raise your legs upwards, straight towards the sky.
- Now bend them backwards behind your head, keeping them straight, until the toes touch the ground.
- The chin will press against the chest.
- Concentrate on the throat centre.

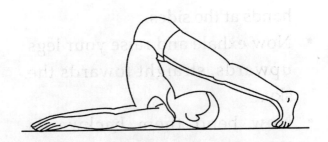

Halasana

64

- One can begin with two to three minutes and increase the time to fifteen or twenty minutes gradually.

Benefits

Indigestion, thyroid, premature ageing, cough and asthma, blood impurities, liver, throat, weakness in the semen, and the problems related to nerves are all taken care of, and a marked improvement is seen in each of these areas.

This posture is recommended for everyone except pregnant women.

The backbone becomes flexible, smartness, inspiration, and delayed ageing are the other benefits.

The flow of semen is reversed and the pelvic region is strengthened. It also helps in solving the irregularities of the pancreas and appendix. Continued practise tends to awaken the throat centre.

Chakrasana

The literal meaning of this word is "the posture in the form of a *chakra* or circle".

Method
- Lie down on a cushion with your face up.
- Keep your feet firmly on the ground.
- Bend the knees and turn the two hands towards the head. Place them on the ground. The distance between the feet, and the palms respectively, should be about

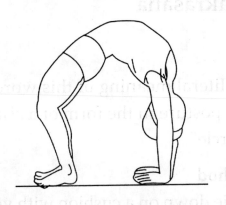

Chakrasana

one-and-a half feet. Now raise the whole body resting on the feet and the hands so that it assumes the form of a circle.

- Respiration should be normal, concentration should be at the navel centre and the eyes may either be closed or open. One can practise this asana for one to five minutes.

Benefits

The whole spinal column and the related nerves are exercised and purified, helping in the awakening of the chakras.

Most of the organs of the body, right from head to toe, are exercised and made strong.

Arthritis and indigestion are cured and the ageing process gets arrested.

Shavasana

The literal meaning of this word is "the posture in the form of a dead body". This is the asana which should be done at the end of all other asanas. Along with other advantages, it brings back the normal flow of blood which was disrupted by the practise of the asanas.

Method
- Lie down on a cushion with your legs spread out.

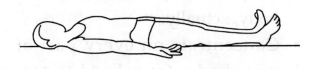

Shavasana

- Your hands should also be kept slightly away from the main body.
- The palms should be open and facing up, your head should face upwards with the eyes closed.
- Keep the body loose like a dead body, actually.
- Concentrate on every part of your body, from head to toe, consciously.
- Withdraw attention from all worldly matters and feel your body relax.
- There should be no tension in any part of the body and you

should feel that each part is getting relaxed.

- Complete the cycle and bring your attention back to your feet. So far, the procedure is enough for the achievement of good health.

  Advanced postures are meant for the more serious students of yoga.

- Respiration should be normal, it should be longer and deeper, and the equal duration of inhaling and exhaling induces concentration of the mind.

- There is a possibility of falling asleep while practising this asana, which should be checked. Respiration should be done for about 5 minutes.

Benefits

Tiredness is removed from every part of the body and one gains strength.

The nervous system and the mind gets rejuvenated. The flow of blood is normalised. The power and level of concentration increases.

Three locks (tribandh)

Moolbandh (Root lock)

Sitting on a cushion, press the root position below the genitals with the left heel. Place the right heel above the left one pressing the point above the genitals. Squeeze the anus muscles and pull it in and upwards. Hold the position. This is called root lock.

Benefits

Rejuvenation of the body, strengthening of semen and observance of celibacy, entrance of *prana* (life force) in the central nerve *sushumna*, curing of indigestion, blackening of hair, hearing the unstruck sound and help in the perfection of "yoga" are the advantages of this posture, if practised regularly.

Uddiyanbandh (Navel lock)
Sitting on a cushion, exhale completely. Squeeze the stomach and pull it in and upwards. The navel region and the intestines will be pressed towards the back. Hold position. This is the navel lock.

Benefits
Rejuvenation, helps in observing celibacy, exercises the stomach and cures indigestion, health, and an

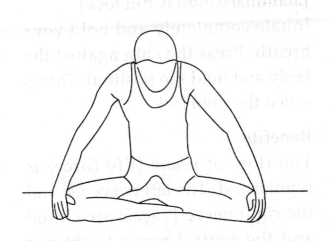

Uddiyanbandh

improvement in the working capacity are the other advantages of this posture.

Jalandharbandh (Chin lock)

Inhale completely and hold your breath. Press the chin against the body and hold the position. This is called the chin lock.

Benefits

The flow of *prana* (life force) is regularised. The left nerve *Ida* and the right nerve *Pingala* are closed and the central nerve *Sushumna* comes into operation, and nectar emanates through the navel, making the stomach healthy.

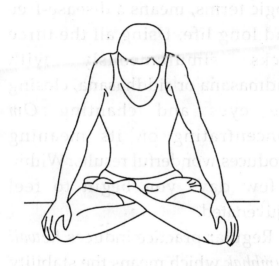

Jalandharbandh

Comments

Each one of the three locks is said to provide immortality, which, in yogic terms, means a disease-free and long life. Using all the three locks simultaneously with padmasana or siddhasana, closing the eyes and chanting *Om* concentrating on its meaning produces wonderful results. Within a few days you begin to feel rejuvenated.

Regular practice induces *Kewali Kumbhak* which means the stability of *prana*, without the inhaling and exhaling practises. When this happens, you achieve perfect health, cheerfulness, you shed extra fat and look thinner, *Kundalini* and *Bindu Chakra* (in-between the eyebrow and crown centre) awakens. One attains victory over the five enemies which are, lust, anger, attachment, greed and ego and the way to your liberation is opened.

On the awakening of Bindu, the nectar flows from it, which rejuvenates the body of the yogi, who then looks much younger than his actual age. The personality of the yogi acquires a sort of magnetism and people are naturally attracted to his discourse as if they are spellbound.

Three Purifications

The Head (method)

- In a broad-rimmed vessel, take one litre of lukewarm water and dissolve ten grams of salt in it.
- Dip your nose in the water and breathe in the water through the nose. Let the water flow out through the mouth in a continuous manner. Take care that you do not breathe in air with water which can set off coughing.
- After finishing the vessel full of water, in this manner, stand up

and breathe out all traces of water left within. The process may appear difficult in the beginning but slowly it will become easy and comfortable.

Benefits

A sort of poisonous fluid flows out of the head which can adversely affect the eyesight, the hearing, and the functioning of the throat. Through the above process called *jalneti*, this poisonous material flows out of the body.

With regular practise one finds an improvement in the eyesight and the process of hearing. Chances of cold and flu are reduced considerably, and one develops a feeling of freshness and cheerfulness. Several other diseases connected with the head are also cured.

The stomach (method)
- Take two litres of lukewarm water and dissolve twenty grams of salt in it. Now sit on your toes and go on drinking the water, glass after glass till you are full.
- Now put two fingers into the mouth and vomit out all the water that you drank.

- Rest for a while. After about an hour, you can eat some rice and lentils cooked together.

Benefits

Those suffering from acidity and indigestion will get relief with this procedure called *gajkarni*.

The process can be repeated once a week in the beginning and then once a month or once in six months. This would suffice to keep the stomach in perfect health.

Problems related to the skin, cough, tongue, throat and chest are relieved.

The body (method)
- Drink 250 grams of boiled but lukewarm cow's milk in the morning, say around 8 o'clock. Rest for about 45 minutes and then drink some milk again.
- Physical labour should be minimised. One should be aware of the incoming and outgoing breath.
- Repeat the mantra *"so"* while inhaling and *"ham"* while exhaling. *"Soham"* means *"I am that"*.
- Consume as much milk as you can digest till the evening. Live on this milk diet for forty days.

- On the 40th day take some juice, soup and fruits, and light rice pudding at night. During this whole process, one should abstain from tobacco, alcohol and sex.

Benefits

The whole body is cleansed and made healthy, smart and shapely.

New blood formation takes place and the power of mind is tremendously increased.

Integral Path in Modern Age

Many postures of Hatha Yoga described in the text may appear difficult to some people, especially those in the middle age. Moreover, many postures are only repetitions and a short-listing is necessary. Also, some people develop problems with the backbone and they need the help of a yoga-therapist. With all this in view, the following set of yoga postures is presented, which is the result of two decades of regular practise. Some of the asanas have been prescribed by Dr Kylee, London School of Naturopathy, and Dr Kiree, University Hospital, Zimbabwe University. The set improves the strength of the back bone; provides all round physical, mental and emotional development; and prepares the person for spiritual awakening, if practised regularly.

Posture 1

Stand straight with a comfortable gap of half to one feet between the two feet. Inhale deeply and bend down at the waist with the two hands resting on the two hips. Remain in the position for four to five seconds and then return to normal standing position, exhaling slowly. Repeat the process ten times.

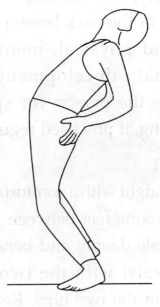

Posture 1

Posture 2

Stand straight with a comfortable gap of about two to three feet between the two feet. Inhale deeply and bend

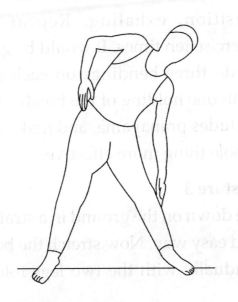

Posture 2

down to either left or right with the right or left hand on the hip and the other hand going below the knee. The bending should be done with a swift jerk. Return to the normal position, exhaling. Repeat the exercise ten times. It would be good to do three bendings on each side with one holding of the breath. This includes pranayama, and makes the whole thing more effective.

Posture 3

Lie down on the ground in a straight and easy way. Now stretch the body gradually with the two legs folded up and the hands drawn backwards. Remain in the position for about half a minute.

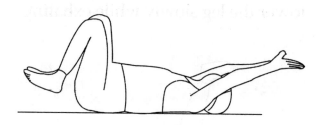

Posture 3

Posture 4

Lie down straight on the ground with face downwards and the hands parallel to the body. Inhale slowly and raise the right leg up to about 45 degrees. Remain in the position for about four to five seconds and then lower the leg slowly while exhaling.

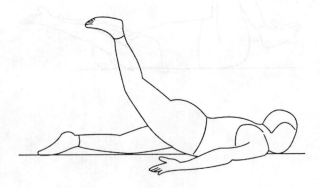

Posture 4

Now do the same exercise with the other leg. Repeat the process six times.

Posture 5

Lie down on the ground with the face downwards, the feet joined and hands parallel to the body. Inhale slowly and raise both the legs together to an angle of about 30

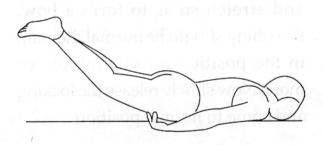

Posture 5

degrees. Remain in the position as long as you can, and then lower the legs slowly while exhaling. Repeat the process three times.

Posture 6

Lie down on the ground with the face down, the legs joined and the hands parallel to the body. Take the hands backwards, hold the feet with hands and stretch so as to form a bow. Breathing should be normal. Remain in the position for one minute or more. Now slowly release the locking and come to normal position.

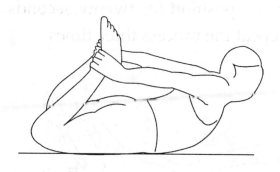

Posture 6

Posture 7

Lie down with the face down. Bring the two hands and place the palms in level with the shoulders. Now raise the head upwards and look at the sky. Take care that the navel region is touching the ground.

Breathing should be normal. Remain in the position for twenty seconds. Repeat the process three times.

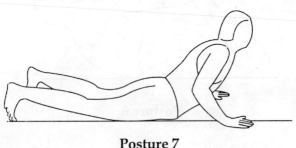

Posture 7

Posture 8

Sit on the ground with your back straight. Fold the legs inside and hold the feet with the palms. Pull the feet inwards so that the heels are touching the main body. Look straight and keep the concentration in the position of the third eye between the eyebrows. Breathing should be normal. Remain in the position for one minute or more.

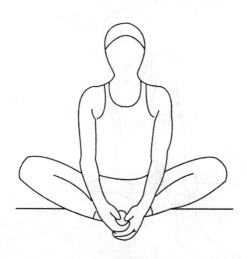

Posture 8

Posture 9

Sit on the ground with a straight back. Fold the right leg in so that the heel touches or presses against the body. Put your left leg across the knee of the right leg in an upright

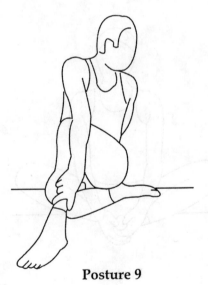

Posture 9

position. Bring your right hand across the left leg and hold the left foot with the right hand. Take your left hand behind the back and turn your head towards the left shoulder, as much as you comfortably can. Remain in the position for half a minute. Breathing should be normal. Now unlock the position, and repeat the process by reversing the role of right and left legs and hands.

Posture 10

Sit in vajrasana by folding the legs and sitting on the heels. Place your hands on the knees. The body should be straight and you should look in front. Take a deep breath, keep the head still, and look to your left as far as the pupils of the eyes can take. Hold for two seconds and then look to the right, as far as the pupils can go. Again look to the left and repeat

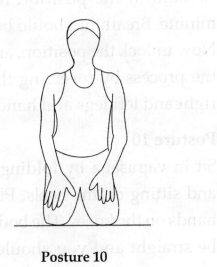

Posture 10

the whole process six times to the left and six times to the right in one holding of the breath. Now slowly release the breath and exhale.

Posture 11

Keep sitting in vajrasana and the whole exercise should now be repeated by looking up, as much as the pupils can go, and then looking down, as far as the pupils of the eye can go. The head should remain fixed and the six eye exercises should be done in one holding of the breath. Now release the breath and exhale slowly. Next, inhale and rotate the eyes clockwise six times in one holding of the breath. To facilitate the movement of the eyes, you can stretch your hand and raise a finger, rotate it clockwise and keep looking at the finger for six rotations. Release

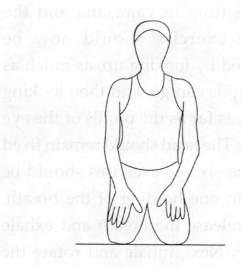

Posture 11

the breath slowly, breathe in again, and rotate the eyes now six times in an anti-clockwise direction. After six rotations, release the breath slowly and relax. It improves the eyesight.

Posture 12

Sit in vajrasana, keep the back straight and focus your attention on the navel region. Exhale all the air out of the body. Now squeeze the stomach in as far as it can go, then release and move it out as far as it can go. This inward and outward motion of the stomach can be performed 25 to 30 times in one holding of the breath. In the beginning, it may be only five to ten times but slowly the frequency will increase. The attention should be at the navel region and the manipur chakra at the backbone just behind

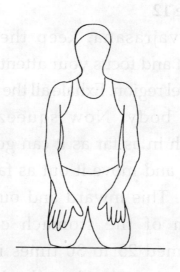

Posture 12

the navel. The exercise is known as *agnisar kriya* and it has a twofold application—removes indigestion and other stomach problems on the one hand, and helps in the opening of the manipur chakra on the other.

Posture 13

Lie down with face upwards, the legs almost joined together and the hands lying parallel to the body. Now, inhale deeply and raise the right leg to form an angle of 45°. Remain in the position for four to five minutes and then slowly lower the leg while exhaling. Breathe in again and now repeat the process with the left leg.

The whole set should be repeated six times.

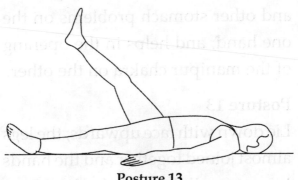
Posture 13

Posture 14
Repeat exercise 13 with both the legs raised together while inhaling and maintain it at an angle of 45°, for about five minutes. The whole thing should be repeated three times.

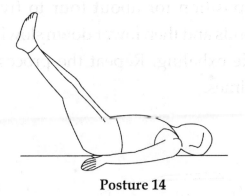

Posture 14

Posture 15

Lie down straight, face upwards, the legs joined and the hands parallel to the body. Now, raise the body upwards from the centre of the stomach as high as it can go comfortably. The body should now be in the form of a bow. Remain in the position for about four to five seconds and then lower down slowly while exhaling. Repeat the process six times.

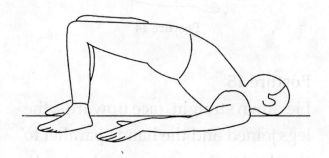

Posture 15

Posture 16 and 17

The exercise is similar to no. 15 with the difference that the hips are to be raised up in such a manner that the body till navel region should be in touch with the ground. Remain in the position for about three minutes. Now lower the hips so as to touch the ground and raise the navel region, making a gap with the ground such that a hand can move in. Repeat the process six times.

Posture 18

Lie down on the ground with face upwards, the legs folded up at the knee and the hands parallel to the

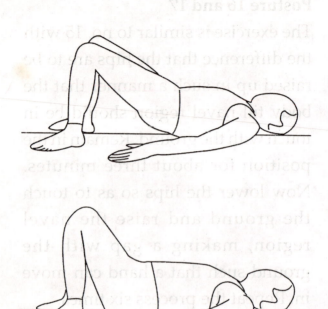

Posture 16 & 17

body. Inhale deeply and turn both the legs together to the right, lowering them slowly till the feet touch the ground. Hold for three seconds and then return to an upright position of the legs. Turn both the legs to the left now till they touch the ground. Remain in this position for three minutes before returning to the normal position. This set of two

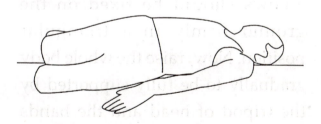

Posture 18

bendings to the right and left can be done in one holding of the breath. Repeat the whole process six times.

Posture 19 and 20

This is "sheershasana" or the head-stand. One bends down over the knees, face down, and the forehead touching the ground. Interlock the fingers of both the hands and take them behind the head. Both the elbows should be fixed on the ground firmly in a triangular position. Now, raise the whole body gradually to be fully supported by the tripod of head and the hands resting on the elbows. Raise the feet

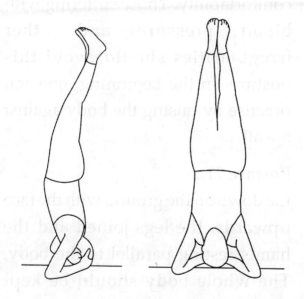

Posture 19 & 20

straight up making the whole body straight. Breathing should be normal. Hold the position for two minutes or more, depending on your comfortability. Those suffering with blood pressure and other irregularities should avoid this posture. In the beginning, one can practise by raising the body against a wall.

Posture 21
Lie down on the ground with the face upwards, the legs joined and the hands resting parallel to the body. The whole body should be kept motionless so that the blood

circulation returns to normal. However, the awareness should be made to rotate from the feet to knees

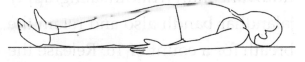

Posture 21

to thighs to pelvic region to stomach to chest to neck to head and then back to feet through the same stations. Motionlessness of the body and rotation of the awareness should be practised for two minutes. This is called "shavasana" or the death pose which rejuvenates the whole system.

Posture 22

Sit in "siddhasana" or in "siddha-yoni-asana". Inhale for a count of four and apply moolbandh and uddiyanbandh while inhaling, apply jalandhar bandh also and retain the breath for a count of 16. Release the three bandhs or locks and exhale slowly for a count of 8 through the other nostril, and then hold the exhaled position for a count of 8. This is one complete cycle of pranayama with tribandh or three locks. It should be practised for fifteen minutes focussing attention on Ajna chakra or between the eyebrows.

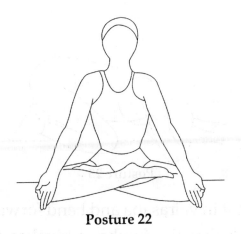

Posture 22

Posture 23

This is "shashanka asana" which is very powerful for balancing the respiration in the two nostrils and bringing concentration between the eyebrows. One begins to feel tranquil which is indeed a preparation for meditation.

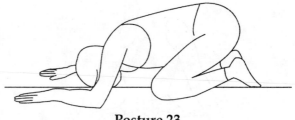

Posture 23

Sit in vajrasana and bend forward such that the forehead touches the ground, and the elbows and hands are resting on the ground. Breathe normally and concentrate between the eyebrows. Remain in the posture for about fifteen minutes. On termination, disengage yourself slowly and either sit in a comfortable couch or lie down on the ground with eyes closed. You can also go into meditation depending on your training.

Posture 24

Lie down straight on the ground with the face up. Bend both the knees and place the palms on the knees. Inhale deeply and then pull the knees towards your stomach in a swift jerk

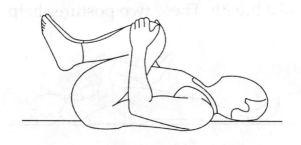

Posture 24

of two pulls and go back to normal holding. Pull the knees to stomach again in the set of two jerks and do it six times in one holding of the breath. Release the breath slowly and lower the legs to come to the normal lying position.

Posture 25

Repeat posture 24 with one leg at a time, doing six pull in one holding of a breath. These two postures help

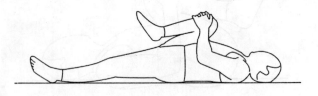

Posture 25

in clearing the gas from the stomach and provide relaxation to the backbone after the set of earlier postures have worked up the backbone.

Posture 26-28

The culminating exercise is now the one for which all preparation has been made so far. Sit in an easy posture with crossed legs or on an easy couch where the body can be comfortably relaxed. An effort should be made to keep the spinal column straight, but neither too stiff nor too slack. Remember that a musical chord instrument, such as

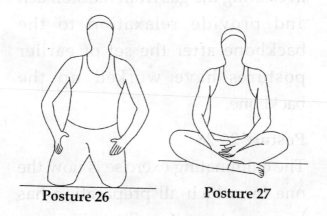

Posture 26 **Posture 27**

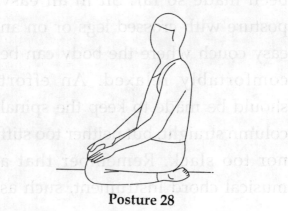

Posture 28

guitar, can give melodious tone only when the chords are neither too tight nor too loose.

Breathing should be normal and concentration should be on the area between the eye-brows or the ajna chakra. Chant *AUM* such that the A begins at mooladhara chakra, U at the anahata chakra and M culminates at the ajna chakra. That is, an elongated chanting of AUM should pass from the root centre, to the heart centre, to the eyebrow centre. This process is meant to arouse the *kundalini* from the root centre where it is lying dormant, and make it arrive at the eyebrow centre where it is supposed to open the third eye or the spiritual gateway to heaven. The chanting should be done for 15 to 20 minutes. At the end, you will find a tranquil concentration at the third eye and you are ready to go into deep meditation.

Now feel that God is pervading the whole universe in the form of Liquid White Light and you are feeling its touch on every part of your body. Just as mercury descends in a thermometre, feel that LW Light is descending on your crown centre and filling the whole body. Bring your awareness to the root centre and feel that a globe of light is shining there. Move your awareness next to pelvic centre or swadhishthan chakra and feel that a globe of light is shining there. In this manner, pass through all the chakras upto the sahasrar or crown centre. Repeat to yourself that all the centres of energy or chakras are open and they are giving their positive power to you.

Now feel that LWL is filling the whole body through the crown centre. Feel consciously that every part of the head is getting filled with Light. Move this feeling to the neck, to the left shoulder to complete the left hand to the end of fingers. Do the same thing with the whole right hand. Now feel that both the hands have become heavier and longer than before. Now move the feeling of Light filling up your spinal column from bottom to top. Next, it is the heart being filled up, the lungs, the intestines, the kidneys, the liver, the spine, the pelvic region, the reproductive organs, the anus region, the left leg, the left foot and toes, the right leg, the right foot and toes. The whole body is filled with Light and surrounded by Light, just as a pitcher in a pool of water has water inside and outside of it. You have become Light yourself by the will of God. The body has become fully immune to all kinds of diseases, decays, imperfections and accidents for the rest of the life.

God is the only doer. We can ask our body to do anything we want, so we are not the body. Similarly, we can ask our mind to think on whatever we want, so we are not the mind too. We are something which is witnessing both of them from time immemorial, from incarnation to incarnation, and that something is soul or *atman* or spirit, which we are. God is the ocean of love and mercy. He has forgiven all our faults and sins and mistakes, if any, and burnt our karmas. We have become pure beings. We can feel the presence of God's hand on top of our head. The rays of Light and Energy are emanating from His hand and are entering our body. Our body is vibrating with his vibrations. This is "shaktipat", direct transmission of energy from God - *Guru* to us.

We will now leave our physical body behind and travel to astral plane in our astral body. Then we travel to mental plane to intuitive plane to soul plane. Here we see Lord Satnam, Master Pythagoras, Lord Sri Krishna, Lord Jesus Christ or any Guru who has helped us so far. Look at His/Her beautiful face. His smile is so pleasing and soothing, rays of Light and Energy are emanating from His deep and beautiful eyes and are entering our body. Our body is charged with his vibrations and we are full of bliss. This is again direct "shaktipat" from God-Guru. We bow down our head to His Lotus-feet.

He is blessing us with His right hand from which vibrations are emanating and entering our body. Our body is vibrating with His vibrations. We will now rise to the higher planes and finally reach the nameless plane of *Brahman* and become one with Him, just as the drop of water merges in the ocean or the ocean merges in the drop. We are becoming the Brahman — *Aham Brahmasmi* — I am that I am. We have realised our permanent Self that is "existence", we are getting intuitive knowledge of the working of the universe, that is "knowledge", and we are full of tranquility and inner peace, that is "bliss". So we have become "existence-knowledge-bliss" or *Sat-Chit-Ananda*.

Conclusion

The above set of exercises is the complete set of an "Integral Path" which can lead to an all round development of physical, mental, emotional and spiritual body leading to self-realization. We have been following this programme at the Academy of Kundalini Yoga and Quantum Soul at various centres in USA, UK, Denmark and Delhi. Many people have reported freedom from the disease they were suffering from, and many have reported good health and vitality. A few selected ones have had experiences with Light and Sound, which are the twin pillars of God. You do not have to take to any other yogic discipline if you take to this "Integral Path."

Special Postures

Gomukha asana

Literal meaning of the asana is "the posture in the form of the mouth of a cow", which is so because the hands joined together at the back give the appearance of the cow's mouth.

Method

It can be done either in sitting or standing position. Raise one hand and bring it behind the shoulder. Bend the other hand and bring it behind the back from the waist. Join the two hands through fingers and stretch them by pulling gently against each other. Breathing should be normal and the duration should be small but increased with time. Alternate the two arms and repeat it

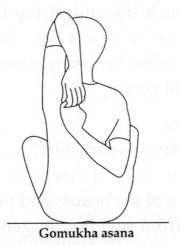
Gomukha asana

a few times, say four to five times.
One will find that it is easier to join

the hands in one position than the other. Some people will find it not so easy to join hands. They should not try to stretch beyond a certain limit and should be satisfied if they can just touch the end of the fingers. Another way is to hold a handkerchief between the two hands and pull gently.

Benefits

The posture is particularly useful for women since it strengthens the muscles of the breasts and prevents them from sagging. In general, it exercises the shoulder joints, pectoral muscles and muscles of the arms. Muscles of the chest are exercised well. An equilibrium results in the energy of the left and right shoulders and arms. Most people have one shoulder lower than the other because of lifting bags, weights or because of playing games with one hand.

Vakshasana

Literal meaning of the word is "posture of the thorax".

Method

Lie down with your face down, arms folded on both sides and palms touching the ground. The level of hands and chin should nearly be the same. Initially, chin is on the ground. Inhale slowly and raise the head and

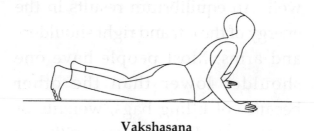

Vakshasana

take it as far as it can go. The pressure is borne by the elbows and forearms. The breath should be retained as you hold the head back. Now exhale slowly and bring your head down. Resting for a few seconds repeat the process. The exercise should be repeated for about 10 times. Concentration should be on the movement and synchronised with the breathing.

Benefits

The posture is very useful for the throat and chest. The larynx is energised and strengthened. It is particularly helpful for those who have to speak for long hours continuously. The lungs are also exercised partly.

Tadasana

The literal meaning of the posture is "form of mountain".

Method

Stand straight with two feet together and big toes, heels and ankle bones touching each other. Keeping the knees straight pull the thigh muscles up, extend the spine and lift the front of the body. Pull the shoulders back and let the arms hang freely. Keep the palms facing the hips with relaxed

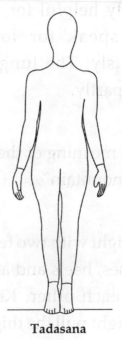

Tadasana

hands. Extend the neck up, relax the face and keep looking straight. Balance the weight of the body evenly on the feet and extend the right and left sides of the body evenly. Practise the posture for half to one minute.

Benefits

It centres the body and brings the energies of the body and mind into equilibrium gradually. With regular practise the body takes a balanced shape and the mind experiences tranquility and peace. It is also a preparation for advanced postures.

Garudasana

The literal meaning is the "posture of eagle". It concerns the diseases of the limbs. Rheumatic disorders of the legs and arms are common things these days. Rheumatic arthritis is a

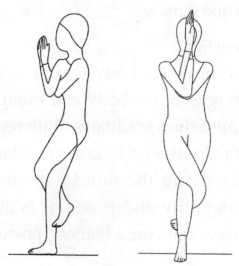

Garudasana

chronic disease of unknown origin which causes disablement and inflammation. Not only the joints but other tissues of the body, such as eyes, pleura, pericardium, lungs, kidneys, etc., may also be affected. The disorder can be either severe or chronic. If it is severe, one has pain, inflammation and fever. No yogasana is recommended in such a situation. However, when the disease is suppressed with drugs, it becomes chronic, there is no pain, inflammation or fever, and yogic postures are useful. The root cause of these disorders is "digestive disorders" of the past. Drugs cure constipation but the poisonous muck and faeces accumulate in the intestines and erupt in the form of pain and inflammation of the joints.

Method

Stand in tadasana (posture 3). Bend the left leg slightly. Bend the right leg and cross the thigh over the left. Swing the right foot back and adhere to the left calf like the creeper going round the tree. Bend the elbows and bring them to the level of the shoulders. Now bend the arms in a similar fashion, crossing left elbow over the right, thumbs pointing towards the face, hooking the right wrist and palm over the left. Remain in the posture for about half-a-minute. Now repeat the process interchanging the left and right sides of the body. Breathing should be normal. Normally 4 sets should be performed. There may be difficulty with the beginners. They can stand against a wall for support, which can gradually be removed.

Benefits

Poisonous muck and faecal deposits flow out gradually and the muscles of the joints are exercised. Pain and inflammation are reduced. Diet regulations are necessary with the posture. Although the food should be according to the taste, it should be nourishing with high vitamins and reasonable proteins. Avoid cold producing elements, such as cold drinks, buttermilk, curd, rice, etc. Warm water with lime is quite useful. In case of excessive pain, fomentation should be done.

Badh Padmasana

Another posture for curing joint disorders.

Method

Perform padmasana by stretching one leg, folding it at the knee and placing the foot on the thigh of the

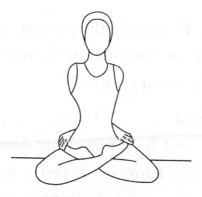

Badh Padmasana

other foot with the help of the hands. Similarly, place the other foot on the first thigh. Keep the hands between the heels one over the other and the body straight. Breathing should be normal. Now cross the arms behind the back, and hold the toes of the left foot with the right hand and vice-versa. Remain in the posture as long as it is comfortable and then increase the duration gradually.

Benefits

Pain and inflammation decrease, constipation is cured and the digestive system improves. The appetite improves too.

Postures for Menstruation

Introduction

Menstruation involves physiological and metabolic changes. Consequently, although it is a normal and natural process, it involves pain and strain. Yoga postures take account of the altered condition of the body at this time and help reducing complaints, such as, backache, stomach cramps, irregularity, excessive bleeding, pre-menstrual tension and scanty bleeding. The following sets of asanas are found to be very helpful.

Supta Vajrasana

Sit in vajrasana. Place a bolster or a set of blankets behind yourself. Holding it against the lower back lie down on it. Put another blanket under the head, if comfortable. Relax and stay in this pose for about 5 minutes and then get up.

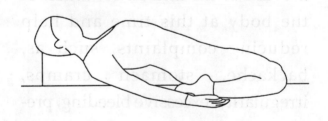

Supta Vajrasana

Supta Baddhakonasana

Sit in front of a wall with the soles of the feet joined together and the knees apart. Bend the toes backward and press them against the wall. Put a bolster behind your body lengthwise, hold it towards yourself and lie down

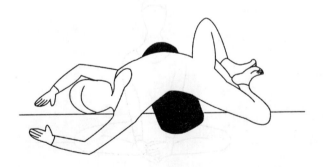

Supta Baddhakonasana

on it, having the shoulders on the ground. Get closer to the wall, as comfortably as possible. Keep the arms either sideways or over the head. Stay in this posture for 5 minutes and then get up turning to the side slowly.

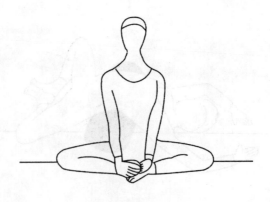

Baddhakonasana

Gorakshasana

It is the 9th asana described in Hatha yoga. Sitting straight, bend the knees, bring the feet together with the soles pressing against each other. Hold the toes and pull the heels to the pubis as close as possible. Stretch the spine upwards and expand the chest. Breathe normally, concentrate on the area between the eyebrows. Stay in the posture for 5 minutes and then release it.

Upavistakonasana

Sit straight with your back against a wall. Spread the legs apart as wide as possible. Straighten the knees and pull the muscles of thighs backwards to the groin. Extend the spine upwards and expand the chest. Breathe normally. Stay is the posture or about 3 minutes and then release.

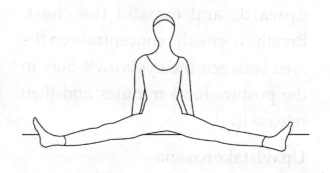

Upavistakonasana

Janusirsasana

Sit straight and stretch the left leg out. Turn the right leg in such that the heel presses against the pubis. Put a bolster across the knee, bend the head so that the forehead presses against the bolster, and hold the wrist of the right hand with the left hand. Put a

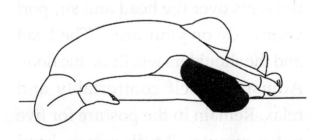

Janusirsana

gentle pressure on the left heel. Breathing should be normal. Remain in the posture for 2 minutes. Repeat the process by changing the side.

Setubandha Sarvangasana
Place two bolsters on top of each other and sit on them. Slide backwards slightly so that the lower back is slightly off the bolsters. Take the arms over the head and support your body on your arms. The head and the shoulders will lie on the floor. Adjust yourself comfortably and relax. Remain in the posture for five to ten minutes. To disengage, bend the knees, push the bolsters away

and align backwards comfortably. Sit in an easy posture and bend forward, resting your head on the bolster support for a while.

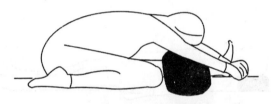

Triang Mukhaikapada Pascimottanasana

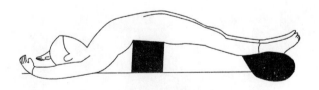

Setu Bandha Sarvangasana

Shavasana

Perform the death posture, (sixteenth posture of Hatha Yoga) for five to ten minutes, turn to a side and get up.

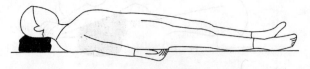

Savasana

General Advice

There are yet more asanas or postures, such as sheershasana (head-stand), but it is not necessary to master all of them. One should select some of them according to one's taste, requirement and suitability, for living a healthy and disease-free life. And, master one of them, preferably siddhasana, for achieving spiritual goals. Knowledge of *Kundalini* and *chakras* and other advanced methods is also necessary.

Hatha Yoga meditation requires more time and application than most people are willing to give. However, a few yogis do practise Hatha yoga as their main method of spiritual realisation. Pure and healthy body, and a clear mind enables the yogi to meditate easily.